HEALTHY...
NATURALLY

EDIMAG
The Popular Publisher

P.O. Box 325
Rosemont Office
Montreal, Canada
H1X 3B8

Tel.: (514) 256-6303 •
Fax: (514) 256-9256 • 1 800 404-4666

Legal deposit: first quarter 1996
Bibliothèque nationale du Québec
National Library of Canada

ISBN 2-921735-17-2

CONTENTS

PAGE

INTRODUCTION 7
WHAT IS HOMEOPATHY 11
A BIT OF HISTORY 13
A CONCEPT OF MEDIUM 17
SUBSTANCES INVOLVED 19
INTRODUCING THE REMEDIES 22
HOMEOPATHY'S HOME MEDICINE CABINET....26
ALLERGIES 28
ANXIETY 30
BRONCHITIS 33
COLITIS 36
THE COMMON COLD 39
CONSTIPATION 42
DIARRHEA 44
FATIGUE RELIEF 47
FEVER 48
HEADACHES and MIGRAINE 50
HEMORRHOIDS 54
INDIGESTION and GASTRITIS 57
INSECT BITES (Stings) 63
INSOMNIA 65
MENOPAUSE 69
MENTAL ALERTNESS SUPPORT 72
PAINS (General) 73
PERFORMANCE SUPPORT 80
PMS (Pre-Menstrual Syndrome)
and MENSTRUAL PAINS 81
SINUSITIS 85
TOBACCO WITHDRAWAL SUPPORT 88
STOMACH ACHES 89
TONSILLITIS 93

WARTS 95
WEIGHT CONTROL SUPPORT 98
CONCLUSION 99

For the purposes of this book, we shall look at some common health disorders that respond fairly well to Homeopathy. However, keep in mind that a doctor should always be consulted in any serious health situation.

INTRODUCTION

While traditional medicine is making constant progress and research into all illnesses - cancerous, cardiac and viral - some patients still claim that this type of medicine does not satisfy their needs and aspirations.

This book introduces you to a form of alternative or natural medicine called Homeopathy, well established in Europe for over a century and more favorably accepted every day throughout America. As a matter of fact, France not only accepts but officially recognizes Homeopathy, and its National Health Plan covers the cost of some homeopathic remedies.

Far from opposing traditional medicine, Homeopathy proposes a different and often complementary, natural therapeutic approach. Its most distinctive feature being a genuine interest in the patient's overall physical condition, it takes any and all individual reactions into account before prescribing a personalized treatment. Evidently, such an approach requires great complicity between patient and therapist.

Therefore, a person deciding to submit to Homeopathy must make a personal commitment. Thus, by identifying with the greatest precision every symptom and possible abuse that could have led to the inconveniences being experienced by the patient, chances for recovery are greatly improved. In fact, to determine the most efficient substance - or substances - to be used, the therapist relies, to a great extent, on information supplied by the patient.

Homeopathy considers that illnesses are the external effects of the body's internal reactions. So, in order to better secure relief for the patient, the therapist must investigate, as far as he or she can, everything that could have contributed to the undesirable condition. All avenues must be fully explored, since the tiniest clue may lead to a remote cause, or remote causes, that have disturbed the system to the point of making it ill.

Since it considers the person as a whole, Homeopathy always investigates the patient's personal reactions to sickness itself, as well as family history (heredity) and physical condition. As I have already said, Homeopathy is a personalized, holistic, natural therapeutic approach, which takes into account the suffering of the individual as much as, if not more than, the pain that he or she endures. Thus, it helps the sick person get better by considering his or her being, at least as much as all of his or her reactions.

This guide will introduce you to a natural and holistic therapeutic approach that has raised many a question throughout the past hundred years or so. Besides showing the advantages and limitations of Homeopathy, it will describe the various substances being used and the different forms under which homeopathic medication can be found, as well as dosages and treatment duration.

This book discusses a variety of diseases, physical discomforts and inconveniences which are treatable through Homeopathy. You must be interested in the subject, since you are showing some open-mindedness about it by exploring this book right now. You are about to discover a natural therapeutic approach which is at once original and human. It is original in that it does not hesitate to depart from the beaten path, and human because it draws all of its power and efficiency from a strong complicity between patient and therapist.

Because, in Homeopathy, the practitioner does not focus attention exclusively on the illness or its symptoms, the patient ends up benefiting from the greater attention he or she rightly deserves.

TO SUMMARIZE...

Homeopathy always considers the sick person as a whole and never limits itself to the sickness alone.

WHAT IS HOMEOPATHY?

To try to define Homeopathy is not an easy task, but its natural therapeutic approach clearly distinguishes it from traditional medicine and its main characteristics can be pointed out.

- Homeopathy considers illness as the body's reaction to external aggression.

- Homeopathy identifies substances which are flowing with the body's natural energy. (A homeopathic treatment cannot help a listless body, because a minimum level of vital energy is essential in order to react and benefit from the treatment.)

- Homeopathy considers the patient as a whole, without limiting itself to illness-related symptoms.

- Homeopathy identifies individual treatments according to each patient's personal reactions.

- Homeopathy takes into account a patient's constitution, heredity and environment, in order to compare and establish relationships between one individual's reactions and those of others who have similar characteristics or symptoms.

- Homeopathy tries to restore a patient's disturbed equilibrium through the use of appropriate natural substances.

- Homeopathy gives primary importance to a patient's own direct information.

THE THREE PRINCIPLES OF HOMEOPATHY

Homeopathy is based on three important principles, which are:

- LAW OF SIMILARS
  There should be a connection between illness and remedy.

- INFINITESIMALITY
  Homeopathy uses vegetal, mineral and chemically-processed mixtures of natural substances, in repeatedly diluted strength to administer minute doses.

- TOTALITY
  Since Homeopathy considers a person as a whole, every treatment is based on the assumption that every illness is the apparent manifestation of a much more deeply rooted disorder.

OTHER FEATURES

Other noticeable points that distinguish Homeopathy from conventional medicine are :

- Physical presentation of the medication.
- Dosage and duration of treatment.
- Substances used.

TO SUMMARIZE...

Homeopathy is a form of natural therapy that treats illnesses with minute, and therefore innocuous doses of certain substances, selected according to the patient's own individuality, reactions and heredity, as well as family and social environments.

A BIT OF HISTORY

Although Homeopathy gained popularity in America throughout the seventies and eighties, it must not be concluded that it is a recent form of therapy.

In fact, we must refer to ancient times to discover its fundamental principles. Some five centuries before the birth of Christ, the Greek physician known as the Father of Medicine, Hippocrates, first wrote that "Equals are cured by equals". Unfortunately, this great medical principle, which means that there should always be a connection between illness and remedy, was forgotten for a long time. However, it resurfaced by the end of the eighteenth century, thanks to a German physician who revived the Hippocratic tradition and became the true founder of Homeopathy, as it is known today.

SAMUEL HAHNEMANN

Born in the city of Meissen in Saxony (now Germany) in 1755, Samuel Hahnemann studied medicine and chemistry before becoming a practitioner. But he soon lost interest in his profession, after noticing that the doctors of his time too often applied drastic and inefficient treatments in severe cases.

Abusive use of practices such as bloodletting, purges, severe enemas and uncontrolled diets, so offended him that he became disenchanted with traditional medicine and abandoned its practice to work as a translator of scientific and medical documents.

This new occupation genuinely excited him, because it allowed him to discover recent and sometimes ancient writings about values, principles and truths which captivated him. Little by little, through his reading and reflections, he came to realize that the medical practice of his day was wrong to ignore certain basic medical rules.

A WHOLE NEW CONCEPT

While still translating documents to earn a living, Hahnemann continued his introspection and finally came to the conclusion that there was a need for a new kind of therapy, one that would incorporate rigorous observation and scientific objectivity.

He could no longer accept all the unsubstantiated statements that came to his attention, even when formulated by the most celebrated physicians of his time. He wanted undeniable proof. His immense curiosity led him to closely investigate many substances. He even went as far as to test them on himself.

Without realizing it, Hahnemann was already laying the foundations of an altogether new therapeutic approach to health that would survive him and conquer the entire world, the one that we now know as Homeopathy, and about which this book is written.

THE LAW OF SIMILARS

Hahnemann continued to conduct new medical experiments, each one more revealing than the previous. One day he decided to try a new substance on himself, one that was being used against malaria, quinine. As he had expected, after absorbing repeated doses of quinine he started developing all the symptoms of malaria.

At the risk of permanently damaging his health, Hahnemann pursued the experiment but reduced the quantities, trying to diminish the negative and toxic effects of the offending substance. The symptoms of malaria reappeared, but with less intensity.

Elated by the preliminary results, Hahnemann repeated his experiment many times, with the same substance and then with others, concluding that:

> **"Any medicine capable of developing the symptoms of an illness in a healthy person can cure a sick person who shows the same symptoms."**

Thus, with proof in hand, Hahnemann reasserted a principle that had already been affirmed centuries before, in ancient times, that :

"EQUALS ARE CURED BY EQUALS"

Thanks to his incredible intuition, based on close observation and sometimes daring experimentation, Hahnemann had simply reiterated a medical principle that had already been put into practice two thousand years earlier by the famous Hippocrates.

WELL-DESERVED SUCCESS

After coming to his conclusion, Hahnemann prudently waited a dozen years or so before making public the results of his research, but they nevertheless caused controversy. After all, he had created so much disturbance by shaking the foundations of the traditional medical structures of his time that he could not avoid controversy. He fought hard to defend his theory and, although at the end of his life he attained well-deserved recognition, nevertheless he was forced to sustain a long struggle.

In spite of events, Hahnemann managed to solidly establish the basic principles of Homeopathy that we still honor today. His doctrine now has many disciples who help advance his resolutely different therapeutic approach by constantly pushing back the limits of the unknown.

INTERNATIONAL GROWTH

Almost two centuries after the death of its initiator, Homeopathy has only recently gained respectability in America. What a great victory for the man of vision who, in his lifetime, managed to make Homeopathy known and appreciated throughout Europe.

In France, where Hahnemann spent his last days, as well as in Germany, Belgium, Great Britain, India, the former republics of the USSR, Canada and the United States, Homeopathy is now recognized as a valid, natural complement to official medicine, one that is able to prevent and treat many benign, acute and chronic illnesses.

TO SUMMARIZE...

Samuel Hahnemann was the initiator, the actual Father of Homeopathy. His research, and especially his experimentation, allowed him to rediscover and reactivate a medical principle, the LAW OF SIMILARS, formulated and put into practice in ancient times by the Father of Medicine himself, the great Hippocrates. From this same principle, Hahnemann advanced the proposition of a new and natural therapeutic approach that was widely circulated and now enjoys worldwide recognition: Homeopathy.

A CONCEPT OF MEDIUM

We have said that the homeopathic approach seeks to be, first of all, a personal one, considering the patient and his or her reactions in relation to the illness. It should also be said that Homeopathy does not hesitate to make certain comparisons and regroup certain categories of individuals, according to heredity for instance.

It is obvious that a number of individuals will observe that their bodies react to abuses in similar ways, inasmuch as they have such things in common as physical constitution, type of heredity and predisposition to illness.

A BIOLOGICAL SUPPORT

These various approaches involve the concept of medium. And, in this context, the word medium corresponds to a biological support which can react in its own particular way under stimulation. This sort of predisposition explains why certain individuals have allergic reactions when exposed to certain environmental elements, while others do not.

The concept of medium, which was first recognized in Hippocrates' time, has been carried over into our modern world and is more than ever alive and well today. As for the definition of medium, Hahnemann himself explains it by defining illness in the following terms :

"We become ill only... when our body lacks resistance and is, therefore, predisposed to succumb to

whichever pathogenic cause is present at any given time."

Now, this notion of medium cannot be dissociated from Homeopathy. It puts the patient in a more global context. It considers his or her particular predisposition to react in one or another way, in a situation where his or her health is threatened.

In this sense it can be said that sickness is the consequence of a disorder within the body itself, and in order to treat that illness, it is necessary to refer to its source. The body has natural defenses that homeopathic remedies are capable of stimulating. Thus, the so-called medium being used is reinforced in such a way that it becomes better able to help the body defend itself against attacking micro-organisms and toxins likely to generate specific illnesses.

TO SUMMARIZE...

The homeopathic concept of medium corresponds to the fact that different individuals react in different ways when an external attack upsets their body's equilibrium and threatens their health.

SUBSTANCES INVOLVED

The best way to discover Homeopathy is to make a close analysis of the substances involved in various homeopathic remedies and treatments. It is also important to understand the different phases involved in the production of homeopathic remedies.

VEGETAL SUBSTANCES

Vegetal substances are definitely the most prevalent among the various ingredients used in the production of homeopathic remedies. Whole plants are usually picked and used at full maturity, that is just before the blooming stage. Sometimes only the flowers, the roots or the fruits are used. Curiously, certain toxic plants sometimes have medicinal properties and, when used in minute doses, prove highly efficient in Homeopathy. The plants used, toxic or other, come from every corner of the earth, from more temperate as well as tropical climates.

As for the manufacturing process of homeopathic remedies, it is fairly simple. After being picked and washed, the plant is cut and dried, after which it is sent to a laboratory, submitted to numerous controls and macerated in alcohol for at least three weeks. Finally, the resulting liquid is filtered to produce a juice called "Mother Tincture", from which dilutions are made.

But the production chain does not stop there. The dilutions thus obtained are then included in different preparations, such as drops, granules and globules.

MINERAL SUBSTANCES

Mineral substances are also natural products. For instance, there are calcium (extracted from oysters) and sea salt, phosphorus, arsenic (that's right!) and sulphur, described as simple elements, as well as composite elements such as sodium salts, potassium salts and caustic soda.

These are only a few examples from among the many mineral products regularly used in homeopathic remedies. However, new substances are being selected, experimented tested every day.

OTHER SUBSTANCES

Besides substances extracted from vegetal and mineral sources, Homeopathy also uses products of microbial origin, vaccines, and even some human secretions and excretions. These biotherapeutic products generally complement other so-called natural substances.

Finally, depending on the presumed cause of illness, Homeopathy sometimes uses other made-to-measure preparations. Special products are sometimes tailored to special cases. For instance, blood, urine or other substances may be taken from the patient and used in the preparation of some very specific homeopathic remedies. Other so-called auto-isopathic blends are also derived from external substances, deemed to have - or suspected of having - caused the patient's illness, such as dust, hair, etc.

Having referred to substances of all sorts, it is now worth repeating that in Homeopathy, all substances and remedies are administered in minute doses, so minute that any danger of contamination, side effects or complications are totally inexistent.

TO SUMMARIZE...

Homeopathy transforms vegetal, animal and mineral substances to produce its medications, and, occasionally it can also use substances of microbial origin, vaccines and other products.

INTRODUCING THE REMEDIES

Substances from which homeopathic remedies are produced are drastically changed before being sold to the public.

From a basic Mother Tincture, also called "Herbal Extract", a final product only emerges after going through several essential stages.

DILUTION

According to serious proponents of Homeopathy, it is only from this essential process that homeopathic medication draws its potency. Homeopaths correctly maintain that, contrary to many allopathic - traditional medicine - remedies, homeopathic remedies can cure sick bodies without toxicity.

I must underline the fact that many levels of dilution meet the diverse needs of patients. A competent homeopathic therapist knows exactly how to administer the proper level to respond to a patient's individual and specific situation.

DYNAMIZATION

When manufacturing homeopathic remedies, each dilution is dynamized. In simpler terms, this means that every time a substance or mixture's original strength is reduced one hundred times through dilution, the flask containing it is mechanically shaken by specially designed appliance.

This operation is absolutely essential to Homeopathy because, while making the product homogenous, it also potentializes its energy. Should this particular stage of production be omitted, any homeopathic medication would be completely ineffective.

Dynamization is what makes homeopathic remedies active. The active agent within any diluted substance is only released and made available by shaking it in a solvent, through the process known as dynamization.

GRANULES, GLOBULES AND OTHER FORMS

Homeopathic medication is commercially offered in specialized health shops or drugstores under a variety of forms. For instance, one can purchase homeopathic remedies in the form of granules or globules, as well as drops and suppositories.

There are also syrups, ovules (small egg shapes) and different tablets and ointments. A patient should seek help from his or her homeopathic specialist in order to choose correctly from the wide selection available.

On the other hand, in order to maintain the potency and freshness of these products, it is very important to store them properly. They need protection against light, high temperatures and humidity, and after use, are best stored in a small kit or bag.

One last recommendation. Avoid opening a tube or any other container of homeopathic medication in a room where perfumes or strong odors are present. And needless to say, keep homeopathic medication away from any cigarette smoke.

TO SUMMARIZE...

The preparation of homeopathic remedies is a process that consists mainly in the dilution of medicinal substances within which, through dynamization, active and curative agents are released.

When ready, homeopathic medication is sold to the public through local stores, in various forms including :

- granules
- globules
- drops
- ovules
- syrups
- tablets
- ointments
- suppositories

HOMEOPATHY'S HOME MEDICINE CABINET

Once you have decided to take advantage of the benefits of Homeopathy and to take care of your own - or your family's - every minor or major illness, you might want to keep a homeopathic medicine cabinet right in your home. This is an excellent idea, as long as you consult a qualified person before choosing the various substances that should be part of your cabinet, the ones that you should, and intend to, keep on hand permanently.

Your health professional will gladly advise you on purchasing, storing and administering these homeopathic remedies, as well as on dosages, duration of treatment and any other useful information. For instance, he or she will probably recommend avoiding high dilution levels to cure minor everyday inconveniences, and advise low or medium dilution levels in such cases.

At this point, being properly informed and having an adequate arsenal at your disposal in your personal homeopathic medicine cabinet, you will be ready and able to respond quickly and efficiently to any minor incident or accident occurring in your home (especially with young children), such as falls, contusions, headaches, colds, flu, etc.

And, of course, in any first-aid situation or treatment do not hesitate to see a doctor if you are dissatisfied with or worried by the evolution of the illness or injury, as you would in any serious situation.

Finally, here is an important piece of advice. Our western world often has a tendency towards overconsumption of medicinal products, so keep in mind that moderation is always the better course of action, with homeopathic substances as well as with allopathic medication.

• ALLERGIES •

People suffer from different levels of allergies. They react favorably or unfavorably to their environment.

WHAT YOU SHOULD KNOW

The causes of allergies are both numerous and diverse, which means that identifying them can often be a difficult task, requiring skin or laboratory tests. And, if allergies return on a cyclical basis, fundamental treatment is a must.

WHAT THEY FEEL LIKE

Allergies take on different forms:

- at skin level they can show up as: • Hives
  or • Eczema

- in the head and chest area they can show up as:
  • Hay Fever
  • Coughs
  • Sinusitis
  or • Asthma

- and internally (in the gastro-intestinal tract) they can show up as: - Gastritis
  or - Colitis

ENLIGHTENED ADVICE

Overwhelming symptoms of an acute phase of apparent allergy, of whatever origin, must be given immediate professional attention. However, relief from inconveniences suspected of being of an allergic nature can be sought from a variety of excellent homeopathic formulations, such as:

- Allium cepa (Onion) relieves nasal and eye inflammation, harsh bouts of sneezing and a tickling feeling in the ears.

- Aralia racemosa (Spikenard) helps relieve colds.

- Arsenicum album (Arsenious oxide) helps relieve coryza and hay fever.

- Cuprum metallicum (Copper) helps relieve sporadic coughing.

- Nux vomica (Poison nut) helps relieve frequent sneezing attacks, nighttime nasal constipation and daytime runny noses.

- Sabadilla (Cevadilla seeds) helps relieve sneezing.

- Sticta pulmonaria (Lungwort) relieves a stuffy, dry nose and a constant need for nose-blowing.

• ANXIETY •

It happens to all of us. At one time or another, we all go through periods of worry and fear. And quite often, these times of confusion and insecurity become sufficiently unbearable to require immediate attention.

WHAT IT FEELS LIKE

A high level of anxiety may trigger many misleading physiological or psychological reactions and anguish can assume a variety of aspects. From a simple feeling of great fatigue, to insomnia, to painful stomach ulcers, physical problems, pains and disturbances related to anxiety are varied and numerous.

WHAT YOU SHOULD KNOW

All forms of anxiety are not necessarily bad, they can also be a source of creativity, learning or motivation. Remember, it might not always be desirable to quell the slightest sign of anguish with some medication or other, or through questionable means.

Make sure you do not fall prey to society's false pretense that any problem can be solved by a pill. Medications for nervous problems may top all pharmaceutical sales, but they are highly habit-forming and too often abused.

ENLIGHTENED ADVICE

As far as chronic anxiety is concerned, Homeopathy has a number of excellent, natural, harmless substances at hand. For example:

- Aconitum napellus (Aconite) can alleviate your morbid fear of dying if you are of a hypochondriacal nature, and especially if you are sick.

- Ambra grisea (Ambergris) is appropriate if you tend to get upset over anything and everything, are paralysed by shyness and constantly afraid of fainting.

- Argentum nitricum (Silver nitrate) helps relieve mild anxiety and apprehension. For instance, if you keep trying to handle every task that comes along, and are always in a hurry and constantly running out of time.

- Arsenicum album (Arsenious oxide) can help if you suffer permanent anguish, aggravated at night because you are afraid of the dark, death and solitude.

- Asafoetida (Asafetida) is suitable for people who are dissatisfied with themselves and irritable.

- Avena sativa (Common oats) helps relieve nervous exhaustion and palpitations.

- Gelsemium (Yellow jessamine) can help if you live as a recluse and have inexplicable fears, if you are anxious over life, death and the future and are extremely frightened of facing people or obstacles, to the point of trembling or diarrhea.

- Ignatia amara (St.Ignatius' bean) soothes the effects of emotions, vexation and bereavement. For instance, if you are very unpredictable and suddenly switch from laughing to crying for no apparent reason, or if discouragement often makes you sigh in despair.

- Kalium carbonicum (Potassium carbonate) is suited for those hypersensitive individuals who dramatize everything and are easily discouraged by the smallest disappointment or obstacle, those people who jump at the slightest sound and react very nervously to the least physical contact.

- Phosphorus may help you if you have constant mood changes, if you oscillate between excitement and depression, and if you suffer from extreme anxiety producing unreasonable fear at the least little problem.

  Psorinum should be tried if you tend to see only the dark side of life, if you constantly seek solitude, and if you eat to compensate for your morose moods.

- Valeriana officinalis (Valerian root) relieves moodiness, nervousness and sleeplessness.

• BRONCHITIS •

Bronchitis is an inflammation of the bronchial lining caused by cold or an excessive use of tobacco. It can generate intense and persistent coughing, morning hypersecretions, respiratory stress related to exercise and variable fever.

ENLIGHTENED ADVICE

For the parent of a sick child, for instance, here are a few particular recommendations:

- Camphora (Camphor) may be given if, after a sudden weather change and a drop in temperature, a child has a stuffy, dry nose.
- Nux vomica (Poison nut) is indicated if in cold and humid air, a child breathes through his or her mouth, has a runny nose by day but a dry nose at night, and if he or she feels better in a warm bed.
- Sambucus nigra (European elder) can bring relief if the child is congested, has trouble sleeping and awakens often with fever and breathing difficulties, soaked in perspiration.

Finally, here are some recommended substances for the relief of the symptoms of the common cold in adults, including congestion, runny nose, sneezing, coughing, hoarseness, sore throat and bronchitis:

- Arsenicum album (Arsenious oxide) helps relieve coryza.

- Belladonna (Deadly nightshade) helps relieve colds, sore throat, head congestion and fever.

- Drosera rotundifolia (Sundew plant) helps relieve coughing and related chest pains, as well as hoarseness.

- Ipecacuanha (Ipecac root) relieves coughing and bronchitis.

- Kalium bichromicum (Potassium bichromate) is used in the case of abundant greenish-yellow mucous secretions.

- Mercurius solubilis (Hahnemann's soluble mercury) helps relieve sore throat, shooting pains in the throat and tonsils, and colds.

- Pulsatilla (Wind flower) relieves a dry cough or a moist cough with expectorations.

IF I WERE YOU

Here are some recommended practices which can help you reduce the severity and alleviate the side effects of bronchitis.

- Curb or eliminate your use of tobacco.

- Avoid sugar, coffee, tea, chocolate, cola and alcohol (including wine).

- Avoid eating sugar-based and flour-based foods at the same meal.

- Keep your liver in good condition.

- Drink herbal teas made from plants which are known to help respiratory functions, such as cherrywood, hawthorn, thyme, rosemary and mint.
- Take effective measures against constipation.
- If constipation occurs, take herbal teas made from laxative plants.

• COLITIS •

First of all, colitis is not colic, it is an irritation of the colon sometimes called spasmodic colitis, or irritable colon.

WHAT YOU SHOULD KNOW

If you are often troubled by colitis, you should submit to a complete evaluation including blood tests, stool analysis, X-rays and coloscopy. You might have a gall bladder problem that needs to be taken care of, but most probably you need to learn to relax and follow a residue-free diet.

WHAT IT FEELS LIKE

Here are some particular signs to help you recognize colitis:

- If your stomach is fully or partly distended.
- If you alternate between bouts of diarrhea and constipation, often accompanied by pain in the lower right part of the abdomen.
- If you have soft, mud-colored stools.
- If you suffer from migraine.
- If your stomach rumbles because of colon spasms.

- If you have permanent or occasional pain along the surface of the colon.

ENLIGHTENED ADVICE

- Aloe socotrina (Aloes) is the proper choice if you have a distended stomach, feel heaviness in the lower abdomen and rectum, emit burning gases and have a recurring need to evacuate, each feeling being followed by heavy perspiring and weakness.
- Carbo vegetabilis (Vegetable charcoal) is the preferred substance if you have some diarrhea, if the upper part of your stomach is distended and pain extends to your chest.
- China (Peruvian bark) is recommended if you have a distended, painful stomach and experience stomach rumbling, with diarrhea and gas. It is also recommended if all food has a bitter taste and you cannot tolerate milk or fruit.
- Colocynthis (Bitter apple) should be taken if. Your stomach is distended, if you have diarrhea and if violent discomfort forces you to bend over to alleviate painful cramps.
- Dioscorea villosa (Wild yam) is recommended if you are experienced violent colic pains accompanied by hiccups, gas, belching and flatulence.
- Nux vomica (Poison nut) is more appropriate if you experience flatulence, have colic (undefined stomach pain) and feel sleepy after meals, and if your constipation involves an urgent need to eliminate with unsatisfactory evacuation.

IF I WERE YOU

You should avoid eating raw vegetables as well as all vegetables from the cabbage family (even cooked) and legumes (dried peas, beans, etc.), green fruit, fresh bread, rich pastries, noodles, prunes, oranges, nuts, french fries, potato chips and purée. As for meats, you should avoid anything with fat or sauce, as well as giblets (organ meats), cured meats, game and snails. Also avoid oily foods, fried eggs, preserves and fatty fish. Refrain from drinking fresh milk, coffee, soft drinks, alcohol and white or rosé wine.

In the vegetable category, the **recommended food list** for colitis sufferers includes carrots, beets, fresh green beans and steamed potatoes (only). Believe it or not, all vegetable (and salad) greens have to be cooked! All the fruit you consume should be either very ripe, canned, preserved or juiced. Dry rusks should be preferred to regular bread, but if you cannot do without bread, make it dry or toasted. Pastries should also be dry.

Noodles must always be cooked in water, eggs boiled and fish oven-baked. You may have grilled or roasted lean meat, cooked ham and shellfish. You may drink tap or flat mineral water, regular or herbal tea, powdered or skim milk, and red wine, but only in very moderate quantities.

• THE COMMON COLD •

We all have experienced the unpleasant symptoms of the common cold and it is obvious that adults can defend themselves against this virus better than children and babies.

WHAT IT FEELS LIKE

Let's say your child is not feeling well, lacks energy and has a runny nose after having been exposed to cold temperatures. This is exactly what is known as the common cold. Nasal secretions that appear clear and whitish before becoming yellowish and then taking on a greenish tinge are sure signs of a viral infection. And a stuffy nose leads to breathing difficulties when the mucus has thickened to a point where it cannot flow normally.

A cold can also be a sign of other types of infections, depending on the symptoms:

- If fever is present you are probably dealing with influenza, more commonly known as the flu, which, with a light dry cough growing into a heavy one and a phlegm buildup, could lead to bronchitis.

- If secretions are mostly at eye and nose levels you are probably experiencing an allergic reaction, usually accompanied by heavy sneezing, such as hay fever, for instance.

- Sinusitis may also be diagnosed if secretions come mostly from one nostril and have a yellow-greenish tinge.

- If the pain is mainly located in the throat, the cold can also be associated with rhino-pharyngitis.

WHAT YOU SHOULD KNOW

When one has a cold, although it is recognized as a passing phenomenon one may want to take a few steps to avoid deterioration of the condition and to try to get rid of it as soon as possible. But before you rush into any action which may be detrimental, here are a few bits of good advice.

ENLIGHTENED ADVICE

For the parent of a sick child, for instance, here are a few particular recommendations:

- Camphora (Camphor) may be given if, after a sudden weather change and a drop in temperature, a child has a stuffy, dry nose.

- Nux vomica (Poison nut) is indicated if in cold and humid air, a child breathes through his or her mouth, has a runny nose by day but a dry nose at night, and if he or she feels better in a warm bed.

- Sambucus nigra (European elder) can bring relief if the child is congested, has trouble sleeping and awakens often with fever and breathing difficulties, is soaked in perspiration.

Finally, here are some recommended substances for the relief of the symptoms of the common cold in adults, including congestion, runny nose, sneezing, coughing, hoarseness, sore throat and bronchitis:

- Arsenicum album (Arsenious oxide) helps relieve coryza.

- Belladonna (Deadly nightshade) helps relieve colds, sore throat, head congestion and fever.

- Drosera rotundifolia (Sundew plant) helps relieve coughing and related chest pains, as well as hoarseness.

- Ipecacuanha (Ipecac root) relieves coughing and bronchitis.

- Kalium bichromicum (Potassium bichromate) is used in the case of abundant greenish-yellow mucous secretions.

- Mercurius solubilis (Hahnemann's soluble mercury) helps relieve a sore throat, shooting pains in the throat and tonsils, and colds.

- Pulsatilla (Wind flower) relieves a dry cough or a moist cough with expectorations.

• CONSTIPATION •

It is such a common condition that many people tend to ignore or neglect it, but any decrease in stool quantity or evacuation frequency can be the cause of lower abdominal pain and discomfort. Not to have any bowel movement for three days can still be normal, but pain is definitely an indication of constipation.

ENLIGHTENED ADVICE

There are several natural substances which can help relieve irregularity, straining, colic pain and flatulence. For instance:

- Alumina (Aluminum hydrate) helps relieve hard and infrequent stools.

- Argentum nitricum (Silver nitrate) helps relieve constipation and dry feces.

- Bryonia (White bryony) relieves constipation that is accompanied by stomach pains which can be aggravated by the slightest movement. Stools are hard, dry and black. This conditions also involves a dry mouth and a thirst for cold water.

- Croton tiglium (Croton oil) relieves constipation.

- Hydratis canadensis (Golden seal) is recommended for people who are constipated because they have taken excessive amounts of laxatives. Symptoms include small, fragmented, hard stools.

- Magnesia carbonica (Magnesium carbonate) helps relieve the frequent and ineffectual urge to evacuate.

- Platina (Platinum) is suggested for those who often suffer from constipation while travelling. Such people often find expulsion difficult, even when they are able to evacuate.

- Plumbum is effective for people whose stools are similar to sheep droppings. They often experience a false feeling of urgency, but evacuation is difficult and may be accompanied by painful anal spasms.

- Podophyllum peltatum (May apple) relieves alternating diarrhea and constipation.

WHAT I WOULD DO

You should never take excessive amounts of laxatives, and any laxatives you use should be mild, such as bran, paraffin oil or Mucilage. Prolonged use of laxatives only encourages constipation. It can even cause colon irritation or diarrhea.

If you are prone to constipation, you should avoid hot and spicy foods, exercise regularly and choose a quiet, calm, regular time each day to eliminate. Also, drink 2 quarts of water and take Magnesium every day.

After about of constipation, increase your fiber intake and eat green vegetables, fruit and wheat bran.

Beware of medication such as codeine, tranquilizers and analgesics, which can also cause constipation.

Finally, if you are subject to frequent or prolonged constipation, you should see a doctor.

• DIARRHEA •

Frequent liquid fecal evacuations may have several causes, such as digestive secretion disorders, intoxications and infections.

WHAT IT FEELS LIKE

There are 4 different types of diarrhea:

1. **Functional Diarrhea:**
   It comes after meals and consists of undigested foods, with diarrhea spells followed by calm periods. Its causes are stress, strong emotions or ingestion of foods not tolerated by the body.

2. **False Diarrhea:**
   Most frequent in constipated people who take excessive amounts of laxatives, evacuation carries the same amount of feces but with a higher frequency. After a "popping cork sensation", very diluted feces and gas follow. This kind of diarrhea requires the same treatment as constipation.

3. **Infectious Diarrhea:**
   Attributed to germs or parasites, it can also follow the absorption of antibiotics. Besides Candida, other germs such as Staphylococcus and Streptococcus can cause this type of infection.

4. **Antibiotic-Induced Diarrhea:**
   Antibiotics destroy the intestinal flora and create an imbalance. At this point, more resistant germs and fungi develop and liberate microbial toxins.

ENLIGHTENED ADVICE

Depending on the circumstances, there are numerous and excellent substances recommended for the treatment of diarrhea. For instance:

- Aloe socotrina (Aloes) should be taken if the diarrhea occurs after eating or drinking and is accompanied by burning and irritating gases.

- Antimonium crudum (Sulphide of antimony) is a good choice when diarrhea comes during a heat wave or after eating certain foods, and when it consists mostly of water and just a few bits of solid matter, accompanied by belching.

- Argentum nitricum (Silver nitrate) is indicated if you evacuate greenish runny feces, accompanied by gas.

- China (Peruvian bark) is the substance of choice if your non-painful diarrhea comes after you have eaten fruit, if you have a distended stomach and the yellowish stools contain bits of undigested food.

- Croton tiglium (Croton oil) should be your choice if you have been taking antibiotics and develop diarrhea, involving the very quick evacuation of watery, yellow feces after the least amount of eating or drinking.

- Ipecacuanha (Ipecac root) is recommended for painful diarrhea accompanied by nausea, vomiting, and evacuation of greenish, frothy or viscous stools.

- Phosphoricum acidum (Phosphoric acid) is more suited to diarrhea that is neither painful nor exhausting, with watery, whitish, odorless stools.

- Podophyllum peltatum (May apple) should be taken if, before evacuation, there is a rumbling feeling and pain, and if, after yellowish feces have been evacuated there is a general of weakness. People affected by this type of heavy diarrhea can get relief from heat or from lying flat on their stomachs.

- Veratum album (White hellebore) should be taken when there is abundant elimination, with cramps and a cold sweat that leave you exhausted.

Finally, if any type of diarrhea lasts more than 3 days see a doctor.

• FATIGUE RELIEF •

ENLIGHTENED ADVICE

Here are some interesting caffeine-free products to help reduce occurences of mental or physical fatigue:

- Avena sativa (Common Oats) helps relieve nervous exhaustion and agitation.
- Medicago sativa (Alfalfa) relieves intellectual and physical fatigue.
- Phosphorus is suitable for people who become exhausted after short periods of physical exertion.
- Selenium metallicum (Selenium) is suitable for people who constantly have a strong urge to lie down or sleep.

• FEVER •

related to the COMMON COLD and the FLU

Fever is a reaction stemming from the body's defence mechanism, which is most often triggered by colds and influenza, or the flu.

WHAT IT FEELS LIKE

When we have fever, we ache and feel stiff all over, we perspire abundantly and we might even shiver. Sometimes skin rashes also appear.

WHAT YOU SHOULD KNOW

Body temperature should be taken in the morning, when lying down. There is fever if the reading is above 100.4 degrees Farenheit, or 38 degrees Celsius.

With fever, as popular belief has it, you should, stay in bed, drink lots of fluids and take Aspirin. If temperature is below 101.3 Farenheit or 38.5 Celsius, no medication is of any use, including Aspirin. On the other hand, if fever rises above 103.1 Farenheit or 39.5 Celsius, you may want to take a cool bath, always making sure that water temperature is no more than 2 degrees Farenheit - or one degree Celsius - below body temperature.

If you wish to avoid some discomfort by staying in bed with lots of slankets on, do so, but not to excess. However, removal of some covers during perspiring spells may be helpful. Finally, it is advisable to drink plenty of water.

ENLIGHTENED ADVICE

When you have a fever, check your temperature closely and regularly and apply proper treatment if necessary. Depending on the symptoms accompanying the fever, different homeopathic treatments may be recommended, such as the following:

- Aconitum napellus (Aconite) should suffice when one has been exposed to cold weather but fever causes no perspiration or shivering.
- Belladonna (Deadly nightshade) is recommended when there is abundant perspiration and when the patient is flushed and feels rundown.
- Bryonia (White bryony) is the appropriate medication if thirst is prevalent and body pain is sufficient to warrant remaining motionless, and in the presence of a dry mouth and strong, heavy perspiration.
- Ferrum phosphoricum (Ferric phosphate) is the recommended substance if fever is accompanied by headache, flushed skin and morning nosebleeds.
- Gelsemium (Yellow jessamine) may be taken if fever is accompanied by significant muscular weakness, chills and shivering, and if there are lapses between perspiring spells and no particular thirst involved.
- Rhus Toxicodendron (Poison ivy) should be taken if your whole body is aching, you are very restless, and if you cough during the shivering spells and have severe rashes.

• HEADACHES • AND MIGRAINE

Headaches are so frequent that they are considered more like inconveniences than ailments by some. However, you should take them very seriously and consult a doctor, especially if there are fever, trembling or vision problems.

WHAT THEY FEEL LIKE

Headaches are usually diagnosed according to where they are located.

Coming from the back of the neck - the nape - they could signal a problem in the cervical vertebrae.

In the facial area, lasting pains usually mean sinus problems. Sudden violent pains - only lasting about five minutes - probably signify facial neuralgia.

And difficult-to-locate facial pains - lasting thirty minutes or so - probably are of vascular origin.

An entirely painful skull - with no other symptoms - could result from nervous tension.

Migraines involve only one side of the cranium, either the right or the left, with pulsating pain accompanied by nausea and vomiting.

Frontal - forehead - headache could result from vision problems, sinusitis or digestive complications.

ENLIGHTENED ADVICE

Here are a few suggested substances for the relief of headache and migraine pain, dizziness and a throbbing head.

- Alumina (Aluminum hydrate) is used in cases of headache where the patient feels as though he or she is being dragged about by the hair.

- Antimonium crudum (Sulphide of antimony) is suitable when the patient has the feeling that his or her head is about to explode.

- Argentum nitricum (Silver nitrate) helps relieve headache-related vertigo.

- Baryta carbonica (Barium carbonate) should be taken if you get a headache with a kind of cobweb effect in the facial area after being exposed to dry cold air.

- Belladonna (Deadly nightshade) is recommended when a headache involves pain that appears and disappears suddenly, that is increased by light, noise loud, and generates a pulsating sensation in the head or neck, as well as for migraines with violent, pulsating pain.

- Bryonia (White bryony) is recommended if you have pain in the back of the head, if it is aggravated by the least movement, and if even the simple act of breathing makes you feel as if your head is about to explode.

- Causticum (Hahnemann's causticum) is recommended if exposure to cold causes a headache and flushed skin, making it difficult to open your mouth, and if it worsens with stormy weather, temperature changes, or during the night.

- Cedron (Cedrone) is recommended if your headache pain reappears every second day or so - often at the same time of day - and is located over one eye, generally the left.

- Cyclamen europaeum (Sowbread) relieves morning headaches, numb headache, migraine during menstrual periods, or headaches with stars appearing before the eyes.

- Digitalis purpurea (Fox glove) helps relieve tension in the forehead - especially when moving the eyes - as well as a tearing feeling in the temple areas or the sides of the head.

- Gelsemium (Yellow jessamine) is for migraine pains extending from the neck to the forehead, with head tightness, sore eyeballs, and preceded by double vision.

- Glonoinum (Nitro-glycerin) helps relieve dull headaches as well as severe and throbbing headaches or migraines accompanied by hot flashes, blood-shot eyes and black spots appearing before the eyes.

- Iris versicolor (Blue flag) is indicated for people with periodical migraines every 3 or 4 days, preceded by bouts of blurred vision and accompanied by acidic vomiting.

- Kalmia latifolia (Mountain laurel) is recommended if your headache pain is located in the right eye or its orbit (socket), and if it occurs abruptly and is aggravated by eye movement.

- Lycopodium clavatum (Club moss) helps relieve headaches where the patient has a tendency to faint.

- Melilotus officinalis (Yellow melilot) helps relieve headache-related faintness and nausea.

- Natrum muriaticum (Sodium chloride - salt) will provide relief if you have chronic headaches with pulsating pain all through the day, accompanied by an abnormal craving for salt, and if you also feel depressed.

- Nux vomica (Poison nut) is recommended when migraine is a direct result of excessive eating, drinking or tobacco use.

- Sanguinaria canadensis (Blood root) is the appropriate natural remedy if, on the other hand, pain extends from the nape (back of the neck) to the right eye and temple, causing hot flashes and a burning sensation in the hands and feet.

- Spigelia (Pink root) may help you find relief if pain extends from the back of your neck to the left eye and temple, if it causes heavy palpitations - especially when lying down - and if you have a fear of pointed objects.

• HEMORRHOIDS •

Hemorrhoids are varicosities of the veins in the anus and lower rectum.

Hemorrhoids can be caused by heredity, lack of exercise, chronic constipation, stress, the ingestion of spices, alcohol or coffee, and excessive effort while evacuating.

Pregnant women are often subject to hemorrhoids.

WHAT THEY FEEL LIKE

Pain, itching, burning and the appearance of red blood, especially following a bowel movement, are common symptoms of hemorrhoids. Complications such as bleeding and thrombosis can also occur, with sudden violent pain.

WHAT YOU SHOULD KNOW

Hemorrhoids are either internal or external.

If internal, they are more often discovered after complications or a medical examination.

When external, they appear as small venous clustersof various sizes, located near the anus.

Remember, thrombosis and hemorrhoids are clots within the veins and they may also be symptoms of other ailments; they warrant medical attention.

ENLIGHTENED ADVICE

Homeopathy has an array of excellent substances to relieve the symptoms of the various types of hemorrhoids.

- Aloe socotrina (Aloes) is appropriate for hemorrhoids that protrude like bunches of grapes, especially if anal burning and itching keep you from sleeping at night and if pain is only relieved when cold compresses are applied.

- Muriaticum acidum (Hydrochloric acid) should be taken if you have swollen, hypersensitive and protruding hemorrhoids and if they are of a dark bluish color.

- Nux vomica (Poison nut) is the substance of choice if you have chronic, painful and bleeding hemorrhoids and if pain increases during the night or while walking.

- Sulfur is recommended if hemorrhoids feel like wounds or insect bites, if the anus is very red and you have burning feet during the night.

IF I WERE YOU

If you are prone to hemorrhoids, be careful not to extend bowel evacuation for too long a time; during expulsion, anal veins become dilated.

Since hemorrhoidal veins are located at the junction of the system that drains the intestine and the system that drains the liver, any congestion derived from liver problems can accentuate the symptoms of hemorrhoids.

Finally, remember that hemorrhoids can be prevented with a proper diet.

• INDIGESTION • AND GASTRITIS

There are many forms of stomach or digestive tract disorders and although they are often mild, they remain difficult to diagnose with precision:

- Simple indigestion, which often occurs after a heavier-than-usual meal, is directly caused by the body's intolerance to certain foods.

- Gastritis results from hyperacidity, often provoked by excessive tension.

- Ulcers regularly result in cramps and heartburn after meals and warrant consulting a doctor.

- Esophageal hernia and other digestive-tract disorders resulting from back problems, anxiety, or cramps due to insufficient exercise also require medicine attention.

WHAT IT FEELS LIKE

Indigestion produces pain in the pit of the stomach and regurgitation, but they are short-lived symptoms that a balanced diet can prevent from recurring.

Gastritis patients feel a burning sensation, commonly called heartburn, which may be relieved by anti-acid substances such as dairy products.

Ulcer sufferers regularly get cramps and heartburn after meals and as previously stated, they should see a doctor.

With esophageal hernia, pain is concentrated at the solar plexus and food is regurgitated. But palpitations and cardiac pains may also be symptomatic of this illness; again, medical attention is warranted.

ENLIGHTENED ADVICE

- Antimonium crudum (Sulphide of antimony) is recommended for people whose digestion becomes difficult after overeating. They have diarrhea, their vomit tastes of the foods they have eaten, and their tongue has a white coating.

- Argentum nitricum (Nitrate of silver) is recommended for anxious and agitated people whose stomach disorders are accompanied by nausea, vomiting, regurgitation, belching and stomach distension.

- Arsenicum album (Arsenious oxide) helps relieve frequent eructations and colic attacks.

- Bryonia (White bryony) helps relieve dyspepsia and regurgitation, especially after meals. You may take it if you feel something like a stone in the pit of your stomach and pain in the upper right part of the abdomen, a feeling that increases when you move and recedes when you rest or apply cold or strong pressure.

- Chamomilla (Chamomile) is indicated when you suffer such intense pain that you cannot keep from complaining, and when you become very agitated and must move about constantly to try to ease the discomfort. You may have one warm and red cheek, while the other is cold and pale.

- China (Peruvian bark) is your best choice if you have a distended and tense stomach, if you feel sharp pain and are unable to tolerate the least noise or physical contact. You may also be affected by painless diarrhea, break out in a cold sweat and lose all of your strength.

- Cocculus indicus (Indian cockle) is the right substance when you are nauseous and vomiting, when you suffer cramps with a pinching sensation and are unable to tolerate movement, cold or physical contact.

- Colocynthis (Bitter apple) is appropriate when you have just experienced a strong emotion or have been exposed to cold, and when you are assailed by violent and acute bouts of pain, which you can alleviate by bending over or crouching.

- Cuprum metallicum (Copper) is a good choice if pains surge like violent and intermittent cramps, if you feel nauseated and anguished, if you have leg cramps during the night, when drinking cold water or bending over provides some relief.

- Graphites (Graphite) is recommended for individuals who feel sustained heartburn and violent stomach pain a long time after having eaten. Often, they are also constipated, feel chilled and suffer from runny eczema.

- Ipecacuanha (Ipecac root) relieves nausea, colic with agitation, and flatulent colic. It is the right remedy for pain around the umbilical (navel) area and sustained nausea, when the patient is vomiting whitish secretions and cannot stand any applied pressure, but when resting can ease the pain.

- Iris versicolor (Blue flag) is recommended for people who experience burning sensations all along the digestive tract, with all foods causing acid build-up and with vomit burning the esophagus.

- Kalium bichromicum (Bichromate of potassium) is recommended for people who have burning sensations that run from the stomach to the spine and experience nausea and heaviness after meals. Their tongue is red and dry with visible cracks, and they may have a craving for beer.

- Magnesia phosphorica (Magnesium phosphate) acts on regular attacks of sharp and violent pain, with trembling and spasms in the hands and muscles. In such cases, some relief is found by applying heat and massaging.

- Mercurius solubilis (Hahnemann's soluble mercury) is the right choice for successive bouts of pain in the upper right sector of the abdomen, which make breathing difficult and are accompanied by foul breath and a whitish tongue. Patients may get some relief from such pain by resting, but they are unable to lie on their right side.

- Nux vomica (Poison nut) is suitable for sedentary people who overwork their digestive tract with large amounts of coffee and tobacco. It relieves digestive spasms, stomach aches and drowsiness after meals. It is also recommended for patients who experience heartburn, nausea and regurgitation, who have a sensitive and distended stomach, whose tongue feels thick and bloated, and who crave alcohol, spicy foods, coffee and condiments.

- Pulsatilla (Wind flower) relieves flatulent colic.

- Raphanus (Radish) is the appropriate choice if your abdomen is distended and the pain only gets worse when you lie on your side, and if your stomach is sensitive to the touch but your condition improves when you release gas.

- Robinia pseudoacacia (Yellow locust) relieves acidity, indigestion and burning sensations in the stomach.

- Sulphur helps relieve eructations, heartburn, and regurgitation of food and drink.

- Veratrum album (White hellebore) is suited for cramp-like pains, vomiting and a cold sweat, with the patient experiencing nocturnal diarrhea and feeling very tired. In such cases, applying heat or taking a walk seem to provide some relief.

IF I WERE YOU

If you are prone to stomach disorders, it is best to avoid spices, alcohol, fats and tobacco. Also beware of certain medicinal products such as Aspirin or anti-inflammatory medications, which can irritate the stomach lining.

It is preferable to eat light meals, even if snacks must be taken in between. It is also recommended to lie down for a short time after meals, in order to facilitate the digestive process.

It is well known that nervous tension often has repercussions on stomach functions. It is important to learn to relax and to release tension by increasing your capacity to express emotions and feelings. There is no better way of avoiding ulcers.

With esophageal hernia, in addition to seeing a doctor, patients must avoid making strenuous effort, bending forward, or wearing clothes with a tight waist.

INSECT BITES

(Stings)

For an allergic person, insect bites can be very dangerous. They can also be dangerous if too numerous, or located on a critical area of the body.

They are generally inflicted by flies, wasps, bees, bedbugs or spiders.

WHAT THEY FEEL LIKE

When a person is stung, there is pain, swelling, and itching in the affected area.

ENLIGHTENED ADVICE

- Calendula (Marigold), Ledum palustre (Wild rosemary) and Apis mellifica (Common bee) may be taken or used in Mother Tincture form to massage the area.

- Citronella and Lavender (in essential oil form), vinegar or lemon juice may be used to treat insect bites.

- Ledum Palustre (Wild rosemary) can be used as a mosquito repellent.

- Tarentula hispana (Tarantula) is suggested when there is significant swelling that is purplish in color.

IF I WERE YOU

In situations where bites and strings are likely, remember, that light-colored clothing is less attractive to insects. If needed, use insect repellent.

If you do get stung, disinfect the area around the sting and if possible extract the stinger.

If the sting victim is allergic or if the sting is located on the throat of near the eyes or nose, seek medical attention.

• INSOMNIA •

No one likes to feel run down all day. Nobody wants to be less productive at work. And who appreciates spending the night with an insomniac child?

WHAT IT FEELS LIKE

When suffering from insomnia, you could have trouble falling asleep and experience frequent and protracted periods of wakefulness during the night.

Insomnia has numerous causes, either related to outside factors - such as the environment - or to your own disposition and constitution and Homeopathy can clearly identify the exact cause before choosing a treatment.

WHAT YOU SHOULD KNOW

To wake up well-rested, sleep is a must. A normal night of sleep is usually divided into 3 or 4 cycles, and each one of these cycles - lasting from an hour and a half to two hours - is divided into the 5 following stages:

Stage 1:	FALLING ASLEEP
Stage 2:	LIGHT SLEEP
Stage 3:	DEEP SLEEP
Stage 4:	PRE-AWAKENING
Stage 5:	AWAKENING

A well-ventilated room, a comfortable bed and fresh bedsheets and pillowcases can create a most favorable atmosphere for a restful and restoring sleep.

Another well-known fact is that physical exercise can induce relaxation, create a healthy tiredness and lead to a most restful sleep.

Drinking warm milk or herbal tea before bedtime is also an excellent habit.

IF I WERE YOU

You should learn to recognize the warning signs of sleepiness. When you feel your eyelids getting heavy and start to yawn, you are entering a sleep-inducing period. And if you should miss it, waiting for the next one is preferable to trying desperately to force yourself to sleep.

If you are oversensitive to external or environmental stimuli, recognize the disastrous effects of stress and learn to relax, adopt new living habits, exclude such stimulants as coffee and tobacco, and make sure the books, magazines and newspapers you read and the music you listen to and the television programs and movies you watch are all soothing and relaxing.

If your children have trouble sleeping, your presence may be of help to them. The time you take to talk to them, to tell them a story or to show them your attention can go a long way towards calming them down.

ENLIGHTENED ADVICE

- Ambra grisea (Ambergris) should be taken if you are an anxious and depressed person and if just thinking about sleep gives you insomnia.

- Avena sativa (Common Oats) helps relieve clinical sleeplessness and insomnia.

- Chamomilla (Chamomile) is very appropriate for so-called spoiled infants who insist on being rocked to sleep especially when they are teething.

- Coffea cruda (Coffee) has a comforting effect on people who are oversensitive to noise or overexcited by coffee. It is specially recommended for those who suffer from uncontrollable obsessions and worries.

- Cuprum aceticum (Copper acetate) is used for the treatment of extreme anxiety leading to sleeplessness.

- Hyoscyamus niger (Black henbane) is used for the treatment of sleep disorders caused by excessive nervous excitement.

- Gelsemium (Yellow jessamine) is suggested if you are easily disturbed major events in your life or if you are frightened to the point of being driven to hyperemotional behaviour, palpitations and internal pains.

- Nux vomica (Poison nut) is appropriate if you are fairly sedentary and occasionally suffer from sleep disturbances, especially after overexertion or a heavy meal.

- Passiflora incarnata (Passion flower) helps relieve sleeplessness.

- Valeriana officinalis (Valerian root) helps relieve sleeplessness in the early part of the night, and as sleep disturbed by constant tossing and turning.

• MENOPAUSE •

This is a natural phenomenon which usually occurs in a woman's life around the age of 50. The body ceases production of female hormones and menstrual periods gradually disappear. A woman is considered to be menopausal when her periods have ceased for more than one year.

WHAT IT FEELS LIKE

The symptoms differ depending on whether the woman is in pre-menopause or menopause.

- During pre-menopause, periods and cycles are irregular and of variable duration. Menstrual flow varies in quantity and some bleeding may occur at unusual times within a cycle.

- During menopause, periods are totally absent and hot flashes, palpitations, and a vulnerability to decalcification have in to varying degrees. Women are often nervous and irritable, and they sometimes suffer from insomnia and depression.

ENLIGHTENED ADVICE

Depending on the particular symptoms and reactions related to menopause, Homeopathy proposes a wide array of substances.

- Amyl nitrosum (Amyl nitrite) helps relieve intense hot flashes.

- Aurum metallicum (Gold) relieves palpitations.

- Graphites (Graphite) is the right substance when menopause brings on palpitations, migraines, hot flashes, varicose veins and leucorrhea, whitish discharges.

- Lachesis mutus (Venom of the American pit viper) helps relieve nervousness, anxiety, dcpression, excessive talkativeness, hot flashes with purplish congestion of the skin and intolerance of tight clothing in menopausic womenwho show signs of distrust, jealousy and volubility.

- Sanguinaria canadensis (Blood root) helps relieve flushes of heat. It is particularly appropriate for women who tend to be excitable and irritable, those who suffer from burning ears, palms, hands and feet, or from migraine on the right side of the head.

- Sepia (Inky juice of the cuttle fish) should be taken if menopause causes pressure in the lower abdomen, hot flashes with vertigo in the morning, and clouded and foul-smelling urine. In such a situation, the woman is often despondent and unsociable.

- Sulphur may be taken when menopause is characterized by palpitations (mostly during the night), hot flashes and burning feet. Often these women have difficulty breathing and feel a constant need for fresh air.

- Thuja occidentalis (White cedar) is indicated for menopausal women with oily skin and a tendency to perspire heavily, to obesity, hair loss, warts or blackheads.

IF I WERE YOU

First, all of your health problems and inconveniences should not be blamed on menopause. They could be of a family, social or medical order. But even if you are in menopause, watch for signs of nervous tension. It may be the real cause of your hot flashes. Stay physically active to avoid decalcification and loss of muscle mass.

Do not hesitate to use cosmetics to fight skin deterioration and always be extra careful with any kind of exposure to the sun.

If the vaginal lining is dried out or if whitish discharges occur, use a topical ointment to supply the necessary hormones, lubrication and protection to fight against infection.

Be especially wary of sex during pre-menopause because of unpredictable ovulation. Use efficient contraceptive methods.

Be aware that hormonal treatments may have their advantages but they can also be damaging. Seek information as well as medical advice and always get a second opinion if you feel the need.

• MENTAL • ALERTNESS SUPPORT

ENLIGHTENED ADVICE

Here are some natural substances to help you think clearer and sharper, without strain.

- Gelsemium sempervirens (Yellow jessamine) can help relieve irritability and the inability to think, or concentrate.
- Phosphoricum acidum (Phosphoric acid) is recommended for people who show general indifference and suffer from diminished mental capacity.
- Picricum acidum (Picric acid) is used for those who show a lack of willpower and suffer from mental fatigue.
- Valeriana officinalis (Valerian root) may help people who demonstrate clouded intellectual abilities and extremely unstable ideas.

• PAINS •

(arthritic, rheumatic, muscular and others)

WHAT THEY FEEL LIKE

This chapter covers a wide range of physical pains with varying causes and symptoms. Here is a list of some common types of pains and brief descriptions.

Arthritis:
Arthritic pains can flare up at the tips or within the joint, or in a surrounding area such as a tendon, a ligament or an encapsulating membrane, when a patient moves. It subsides with rest or a good night's sleep. However, it involves no swelling, redness or inflammation.

Back pains:
Today's most common complaint, back pains are most often caused by traumatism, inflammatory ailments or deformities.

If back pains are due to a traumatism or a deformity, they are generally brought on by movement or effort. On the other hand, if they are of an inflammatory nature they most probably appear every morning, diminish during the day, and reappear every night.

It is difficult to define back pains because the spine itself includes several sections and a problem in one section can have repercussions on another, be it lumbar, dorsal or cervical.

Bursitis:
This serious inflammation of a bursa - a sac containing the lubricating substance of a joint - can occur in a shoulder, an elbow, a hip or a knee and can even lock a joint if calcification is present.

Cramps:
Cramps are simply painful, involuntary and transitory contractions of certain muscles. Here is some useful information to help explain cramps and their causes.

Epicondylitis or Tennis Elbow:
As its name implies, it is localized at elbow level; it affects only one tendon attached to one of the elbow muscles, the epicondyl. This type of pain makes some simple gestures, such as shaking hands, opening a door or pouring a drink, very painful. Pain can be felt down to the wrist, but will subside during the night when the patient is at rest.

Inflammation:
Inflammation of a joint is characterized by redness, swelling and a hot sensation, experienced mostly during late-night or early-morning hours. Inflammation pain cannot be relieved by rest and it reappears again at night.

Joint pains:
The connections between the bones in our bodies can be traumatically attacked, and when this happens there is peripheral or internal pain which can be attributed either to the joint itself or to surrounding areas, such as ligaments and tendons. The joint system is an interdependent network, so

a problem in one joint can create complications in others. The main causes of joint pains are: arthritis, traumatism, inflammation and infection.

Lumbago:

This type of lower back pain is usually not extend into the legs. In a true case of lumbago, pain suddenly appears after a particular movement, effort or fall and it feels like a rigid bar restricting the lower back and making certain movements painful. In chronic lumbago, the pain appears in the morning, disappears as the patient warms up, reappears at the end or the day and can be alleviated by lying down.

Nape (neck) pains:

More frequent in women than men, especially office workers, this pain is mostly located at the nape of the neck; it can also extend into the head, the forehead, the shoulders and the back. The principal causes of neck pains are: calcification, automobile accidents, traumatism, and cervical arthritis. Other factors, such as menstruation, nervous tension, vertebral congestion and back-muscle deficiency, can also result in pain at the nape of the neck.

Rheumatism:

Many types of pain and different problems are covered under this general term, although all of them cannot be confirmed as rheumatic in nature. This is why some types of pains are listed separately and under their own name in this book. However, to familiarize yourself with some of these different manifestations, let's look at 7 types of rheumatic pain.

1 - **Pain that subsides with movement**
This is often the case with sports-related rheumatism. This pain sometimes increases with immobility, cold or humidity and subsides with movement or hot compresses.

2 - **Pain that is caused by overexertion**
You feel stiff and ache all over, to the point of not being able to tolerate even the slightest physical contact; you get relief from lying down, but your bed feels harder than it really is.

3 - **Pain that subsides with rest**
Swollen joints of a dark red color, superficial pain in warm weather and deeper pain when it gets cold is called gout. Often, when joints are red and warm any movement can induce pain and only total rest and warm compresses can ease it.

4 - **Pain that increases with humidity**
Muscles ache and the patient has to keep moving but gets no relief in doing so. Attacks appear and disappear suddenly and pain switches from place to place. Individuals who are on the heavy side, especially at the hips and buttocks, experience cracking joint noises and can only ease their pain by moving very slowly.

5 - **Pain that subsides with humidity**
Characterized by a burning sensation and accompanied by stiff joints and taut tendons, this pain is aggravated by dry cold and relieved by warm humidity.

6 - **Pain that is reduced by cold**
This type of rheumatism usually starts in the feet and progresses upwards. Joints are swollen with a blueish paleness or a reddish tinge, and pain can be soothed by cold compresses or substantially reduced when feet are in cold water.

7 - **Pain that is intensified by an oncoming storm**
This consists of zigzagging pains which increase during nighttime and resting periods and diminish when the patient starts moving or when the storm has gone by.

Shoulder pains:
Various ailments causing shoulder pain are included here. Most often, shoulder pain or periarthritis is caused by tendinitis in one of the shoulder muscles. Pain can radiate into the upper arm, the neck and the thorax, and its consequences vary in intensity, from a simple mobility inconvenience to a total arm incapacity. X-raying the shoulder and neck area may be necessary for diagnosis, and calcification may be involved.

Traumatism:
From an insect bite to severe fractures, traumatisms are lesions accidentally caused to body tissues, organs or limbs. They can result from an impact or a fall and have very damaging repercussions on body joints. Nerve traumatism causes acute pain that radiates along the affected nerve. Cranial (skull) traumatism also causes vertigo, loss of memory or insomnia. Joint traumatism may cause a synovial (lubrication) loss.

Tendinitis:
Tendinitis is inflammation of a tendon, which joins muscle tissue to bone tissue. Muscles are fairly elastic, but when they are submitted to strenuous effort micro-ruptures can occur, especially within the tendons, and this causes pain. It can occur wherever a tendon exists in the human body, but it is most often concentrated in the shoulder, elbow or knee areas.

ENLIGHTENED ADVICE

For effective relief from most pains - and especially arthritic and rheumatic pain, stiffness and pain of the joints, lumbago and sciatica - the following substances are recommended:

- Apis mellifica (Common bee) is used to help relieve finger numbness.

- Arnica montana (Leopard's bane) reduces finger cramps.

- Arsenicum album (Arsenious oxide) helps relieve acute arm, hand and leg pains.

- Benzoicum acidum (Benzoic acid) relieves joint pains and neck stiffness.

- Causticum (Hahnemann's causticum) helps relieve arthritic and rheumatic pain, stiffness of the back, as well as shooting pains and acute pulling in the thighs, legs, knees and feet.

- Colchicum autumnale (Wild saffron) helps relieve gout, finger cramps and pains in the legs, feet and toes.

- Natrum carbonicum (Sodium carbonate) helps relieve shoulder pains.

• PERFORMANCE • SUPPORT

ENLIGHTENED ADVICE

Here are some caffeine-free substances to increase stamina and help prevent exercise-related trauma and cramping.

- Calcarea carbonica (Calcium carbonate) is suitable for strong persons.
- Medicago sativa (Alfalfa) helps relieve physical and intellectual fatigue.
- Natrum sulfuricum (Sodium sulphate) is a nerve stimulant.
- Rubia tinctoria (Dyer's madder) is generally used for disorders affecting the bones.
- Sarcolacticum acidum (Sarcolactic acid) is used against muscular fatigue, pain, swelling, stiffness and tenderness of the joints.
- Silicea (Silica) is recommended for people who lack mental and physical stamina or self-confidence.

• PMS •
(Pre-Menstrual Syndrome)
AND
MENSTRUAL PAINS

PMS appears one week before menstrual periods and is mostly caused by a hormone imbalance, for the most part due to an excess of estrogen as compared to progesterone; Menstrual pains are the symptoms and pains that occur during menstrual periods.

WHAT THEY FEEL LIKE

Women suffering from pre-menstrual syndrome, or PMS, can experience various head or back pains and are often nervous and irritable. They feel heaviness in their legs and pain in the lower abdomen and in the breasts. Their stomach may be distended and their body weight may increase slightly.

During menstrual periods, some light lower-abdomen and lower-back pains are considered normal; if they become too severe, they should be treated as an illness.

WHAT YOU SHOULD KNOW

All pains preceding menstrual periods and recurring on a regular basis can be considered symptoms of PMS.

Of the 5% of all young women who suffer from abnormal menstrual pains, 10% experience with spontaneous relief, another 10% see their pains disappear after their first sexual relation, and another 65% after their first pregnancy.

In mature women, painful periods are due to genital infection, hormone disorders, cervical spasms or endometriosis.

ENLIGHTENED ADVICE

- Aurum metallicum (Gold) relieves symptoms of sadness, irritability and anger.

- Chamomilla (Chamomile) is recommended for intolerable pain, agitation and a black, clotty, blood flow.

- Cimicifuga racemosa (Black cohosh) helps relieve period pains, moodiness and menstrual headaches. It can also relieve ovarian pains during ovulation if the patient alternates between periods of depression and excitement and if her breasts ache and she has a feeling of heaviness in her lower abdomen.

- Colocynthis (Bitter apple) and Magnesia phosphorica (Magnesium phosphate) may be used alternately when there is intolerable pain that begins and ceases abruptly, and for violent cramps.

- Cyclamen europaeum (Sowbread) is good for headaches and may help with vertigo, nausea, and vision problems when the person is depressed and has no appetite.

- Folliculinum (Estrogen) should be taken for any pre-menstrual problem.

- Histaminum (Histamine) should be taken on a daily basis during periods.

- Hydrastis canadensis (Golden seal) helps relieve menorrhagia (excessive menstrual discharge) and metrorrhagia (non-menstrual uterine hemorrhage).

- Hyoscyamus niger (Black henbane) helps relieve metrorrhagia (uterine hemorrhage), cramps and headache.

- Ignatia (St.Ignatius' bean) is recommended for problems such as moodiness or a lumpy feeling in the throat or the pit of the stomach.

- Lac caninum (Dog's milk) is for menstruation characterized by sensitive, swollen and aching breasts and a sore throat.

- Luteinum (Corpus luteum) may be taken from the 15th to the 25th day of the cycle, if results are unsatisfactory.

- Lycopodium clavatum (Clubmoss) helps relieve dispondency and a bloated stomach.

- Mercurius corrosivus (Mercury chloride) in homeopathic dilutions helps relieve anxiety, anger, and periods that are too early and too heavy.

- Natrum muriaticum (Sodium chloride - salt) can relieve pain in the lower abdomen and lower back in a case where the patient is sad and depressed, gains weight and suffers from oedema (water retention).

- Nitricum acidum (Nitric acid) relieves irritability.

- Pulsatilla (Wind flower) is appropriate for individuals - mostly mild, timid and easily given to crying - whose pains are located around the kidney and thigh area, and who have a reduced flow of thick, blackish blood.

- Sabina (Savin juniper) can be helpful in cases of a heavy menstrual flow with violent pains extending from the sacrum to the pubis, and shooting pains in the vagina itself.

- Secale cornutum (Rye ergot) helps relieve anxiety.

- Sepia (Inky juice of the cuttle fish) can help when extreme pressure is felt in the lower abdomen and the individual feels sad, lonely and indifferent.

Oenothera Oil, Borage Oil and Vitamin E may also be helpful, as well as herbal teas made from diuretic plants such as Mouse ear, Olive and Cherry stems.

IF I WERE YOU

Consult a gynecologist, watch your weight and learn to relax. Nervousness can only increase hormone disorders.

Avoid tea and coffee and beware of hormonal treatments, which may create as many problems as they solve.

• SINUSITIS •

Sinuses are cavities located within our facial bones and sinusitis is the inflammation of these frontal cavities.

Its causes are often of an allergic nature and a proper diagnosis can only be made after an x-ray examination.

WHAT IT FEELS LIKE

After a cold, if you feel a warm sensation in the forehead area when you bend down and if you experience persistent yellowish secretions, you may be suffering from acute sinusitis.

On the other hand, if you experience headaches rather than sinus pains it could be a case of chronic sinusitis.

WHAT YOU SHOULD KNOW

If you tend to have repeated bouts of sinusitis, you can alleviate and possibly eliminate its unpleasant symptoms and give your respiratory passages a respite by following these simple rules:

- do not smoke;
- avoid contact with pollutants;
- maintain a reasonable level of humidity in your home;
- and practice helpful breathing techniques.

If you are prone to sinusitis you may also be highly sensitive to atmospheric pressure changes. If so, avoid and beware of flying and high altitudes, as well as scuba-diving and other underwater activities.

ENLIGHTENED ADVICE

Homeopathic treatment of sinusitis varies according to its type, symptoms, and persistence. Here are a few recommendations, depending on the symptoms experienced.

- Allium cepa (Onion) relieves nasal inflammation characterized by discharges.

- Belladonna (Deadly nightshade) may be taken at the beginning of a sinus attack, when pains are often sharp but there is no runny nose although there may be some congestion.

- Euphrasia officinalis (Eyebright) helps relieve inflammation of the eyes and the nose.

- Hepar sulphuris calcareum (a homeopathic preparation of Sulphur and oyster shell) may be taken when the sinus attack is still recent. It helps relieve mucous membrane inflammation and sharp pains, of the type that can be worsened by touching or by exposure to cold air.

- Hydrastis canadensis (Golden seal) is recommended for rundown, emaciated patients with chronic yellowish, viscous secretions that often irritate the nostrils.

- Kalium bichromicum (Bichromate of potassium) is preferable for heavier individuals experiencing strong pain at the base of the nose, with very thick secretions of a yellowish-greenish coloring often crusting in the nostrils.

- Mezereum (Spurge olive) should be taken when sharp pain is felt in facial and nasal bones, and when yellowish secretions are sometimes tinged with blood.

- Nux vomica (Poison nut) helps relieve internal sensitiveness, inflammation and obstructions in the nose, as well as nostril pain.

- Silicea (Silica) may be taken in combination with other substances, if sinusitis is more persistent.

- Sticta pulmonaria (Lungwort) relieves a stuffy, dry nose and pressure at the base of the nose.

- Thuja occidentalis (White cedar) is used for greenish and fetid nasal discharges.

• SMOKING • WITHDRAWAL SUPPORT

ENLIGHTENED ADVICE

Here are some natural substances that can help relieve the craving and frustration of tobacco withdrawal.

- Magnesia phosphorica (Magnesium phosphate) relieves headache and stomach cramps.
- Staphysagria (Stavesacre) helps reduce the effects of tobacco smoking, such as excoriated (peeling) tongue and gastralgia, or stomach pain.
- Tabacum (Tobacco) and Lobelia inflata (Indian tobacco) are choice substances in such circumstances according to a quote from John Henry Clarke taken from the Dictionary of Practical Materia Medica: "No remedy did good until he remained one evening with two friends who were smoking and got himself well-saturated with the smoke... that cured him."
- Thuja occidentalis (White cedar) can help relieve sadness, irritability and depression brought on by the withdrawal of tobacco.

• STOMACH ACHES •

Under this general heading are problems involving the stomach, liver, gallbladder, pancreas, colon and also some back and nervous problems.

WHAT YOU SHOULD KNOW

In the presence of acute stomach pains, hypersensitivity, stiffness at the slightest touch, vomiting, irregular bowel movements, fever or bleeding, a doctor should be consulted immediately. If a serious traumatism, injury or accident is involved, hospitalization is urgent.

There are two possible major causes for most stomach pains: food and nerves. We eat too much and we eat the wrong foods. We are subjected to too much harmful stress. We must adopt good living habits, exercise regularly, and learn relaxation techniques.

ENLIGHTENED ADVICE

Other chapters in this book explore certain related problems in detail. However, here are some substances to use for the safe and effective relief from digestive discomfort, nausea, bloating gas and related pains.

- Arsenicum album (Arsenious oxide) helps relieve frequent belching and colic attacks.

- Bryonia (White bryony) helps relieve dyspepsia and regurgitation, especially after a meal. You may take it if you feel something like a stone in the pit of your stomach and pain in the upper right part of the abdomen, a feeling that increases when you move and recedes when you rest or apply cold or strong pressure.

- Chamomilla (Chamomile) is indicated when you suffer such intense pain that you cannot keep from complaining, when you are very agitated and have to move constantly to try to ease the discomfort. You may have one warm and red cheek, while the other is cold and pale.

- China (Peruvian bark) is your best choice if you have a distended and taut stomach, and if you feel sharp pain and are unable to tolerate the least noise or physical contact. You may also be affected by painless diarrhea, break out in a cold sweat and have a complete loss of strength.

- Cocculus indicus (Indian cockle) is the right substance when you are nauseous and vomiting, when you suffer cramps with a pinching sensation and are unable to tolerate movement, cold or shock.

- Colocynthis (Bitter apple) is appropriate when you have just experienced a strong emotion or exposed to cold, and when you are assailed by violent and acute bouts of pain which you can alleviate by bending or crouching.

- Cuprum metallicum (Copper) is the proper choice when pains consists of violent and intermittent cramps, when you feel nauseated and anguished, when you have leg cramps during the night and when drinking cold water or bending over provides some relief.

- Ipecacuanha (Ipecac root) relieves nausea, colic with agitation, and flatulent colic. It is the right remedy for pain around the umbilical (navel) area and sustained nausea, when the patient is vomiting whitish secretions and cannot stand any applied pressure, but when resting can relieve the pain.

- Magnesia phosphorica (Magnesium phosphate) acts on regular attacks of sharp and violent pain, with trembling and spasms in the hands and muscles. In such cases, some relief is found by applying heat and massaging.

- Mercurius solubilis (Hahnemann's soluble mercury) is the right choice for successive bouts of pain in the upper right sector of the abdomen, which make breathing difficult and are accompanied by foul breath and a whitish tongue. Patients may get some relief from such pain by resting, but they are unable to lie on their right side.

- Nux vomica (Poison nut) will help if you have overeaten and feel pain about an hour after the meal, and if you also feel a heaviness that subsides when you lie down, bend down, or press firmly against your abdomen.

- Pulsatilla (Wind flower) relieves flatulent colic.

- Raphanus (Radish) is the proper choice if your abdomen is distended and the pain only gets worse when you lie on your side, and if your stomach is sensitive to the touch but your condition improves when you release gas.

- Robinia pseudoacacia (Yellow locust) relieves acidity, indigestion and burning sensations in the stomach.

- Sulphur helps relieve eructations, heartburn, and regurgitation of food and drink.

- Veratrum album (White hellebore) is suited for cramp-like pains, vomiting and a cold sweat, when the patient experiences nocturnal diarrhea and feels very tired. In such cases, applying heat or taking a walk may bring relief.

• TONSILLITIS •

This type of inflammatory disorder cannot really be considered an illness. It is the symptom of another physiological problem. Most often a sore throat is due to a virus. Such cases happen to be more frequent in children because their tonsils are their only real front-line defence against infection.

WHAT IT FEELS LIKE

When you have been exposed to cold and the roof of your mouth is ticklish, when you have trouble swallowing because of a reddened, irritated throat, with or without white spots, you definitely have a throat infection.

WHAT YOU SHOULD KNOW

Since very young babies are more sensitive to these kinds of infections, breastfeeding is recommended because the mother's milk is rich in antibodies.

For children with throat infections, the environment should be kept free of any dust or smoke, overheating should be avoided, and rooms should be well ventilated.

ENLIGHTENED ADVICE

Depending on the throat's condition and the evolution of the illness, Homeopathy offers a variety of interesting and efficient medicinal substances.

- Aconitum napellus (Aconite) may be taken if you have just been exposed to cold and feel feverish and jittery, which suggests the beginning of a throat infection.

- Phytolacca decandra (Poke) should be taken if you definitely suffer from tonsillitis and are experiencing general fatigue, with general aches and pains, and if your throat is dark red and you can barely swallow. You should see a doctor if you suffer from sore throat on a recurring basis.

• WARTS •

This type of infection, attributed to the Papova Virus, occurs when the body's natural defences become deficient; it should always be treated.

Common warts are benign lesions found mostly on open skin areas, isolated or in groups. They vary in diameter between an eighth and a quarter of an inch.

Flat warts are generally located on the face, the neck or the back of the hands. They are barely visible since they often have very little color or thickness.

Plantar warts grow on the soles of the feet.

WHAT THET FEEL LIKE

Common and flat warts are generally painless, but plantar warts are painful because of the pressure that is applied when walking.

WHAT YOU SHOULD KNOW

Do not confuse moles with warts. If a mole becomes sensitive, if it grows or changes color, consult a doctor.

Pregnant women should not worry if their warts grow in size during pregnancy. However, warts should be treated, especially if they appear on a part of your body where they can create a problem or a psychological traumatism.

Watch for infection, especially with plantar warts. Remember that once infected, you do not necessarily become immune to further infection from the same virus.

ENLIGHTENED ADVICE

- Thuja occidentalis (White cedar) is recommended for all warts, along with the following substances.
- Antimonium crudum (Sulphide of antimony) should be taken for plantar warts or hard, caloused growths on the inside of the hands of patients who have a whitish tongue and digestive problems.
- Causticum (Hahnemann's causticum) should be taken for warts with an irregular appearance, that bleed and are sensitive to the touch, and that are located under the fingernails or on the nose.
- Dulcamara (Bittersweet) is effective against flat warts on the back of the hands, as well as wide soft, brown, translucid warts that often grow on the back.
- Natrum sulfuricum (Sodium sulphate) is more appropriate for warts that are aggravated and made more sensitive by humidity, and that are located on the scalp, the face, the eyelids, the breasts or the genitals.

- Nitricum acidum (Nitric acid) is indicated for hard, calloused warts of a yellowish, golden color, or those with painful and sometimes bleeding cracks.

IF I WERE YOU

Before submitting to any radical treatment, remember that there may be less drastic methods that are worth trying.

• WEIGHT • CONTROL SUPPORT

ENLIGHTENED ADVICE

If you are trying to control your weight or if you are simply weight-conscious, the following substances can help you increase your metabolic rate, reduce bloating and improve digestion.

- Fucus vesiculosus (Sea kelp) is used to fight against obesity and to improve digestion.
- Kalium iodatum (Potassium iodide) can help control the type of hunger that increases one day and diminishes the next.
- Rhamnus frangula (Buckthorn) is a non-irritating laxative to be used against obesity and cellulitis.
- Thyroidinum (Thyroid extract in homeopathic dilutions) can help increase your metabolic rate.

CONCLUSION

Through this book, I have helped you understand a form of alternative, natural, holistic medicine called Homeopathy. You have learned that this different, complementary therapeutic approach has been practised in Europe for over a century and is rapidly gaining ground in America.

By describing many specific diseases, symptoms, physical discomforts and inconveniences, all treatable through Homeopathy, and by mentioning substances used in treatments, the forms under which medications are found, the dosages and treatment durations, and by generally showing a realistic picture of the limitations as well as the advantages of Homeopathy, I sincerely hope that I have made you more aware of the importance of physical health and given you new knowledge and better means to achieve well-being.

I have also tried to show you how, through the use of its natural, harmless substances and its exclusive formulas, Homeopathy has as much potential for preventing illness as it has for restoring and maintaining a healthy equilibrium.

Allow me to emphasize the fact that Homeopathy is not only original - in that it does not hesitate to depart from the beaten path - but very human. It always considers the the person as a whole instead of limiting itself to the illness, which is only an external consequence of the body's internal reactions.

I hope that now that you have read this book, you will look for more information on Homeopathy. Take good care of yourself and enjoy a long, happy and healthy life.